Ginger's 15 Minute Mindfully Aligned Morning Workout
Photos by Deb Foster Photography

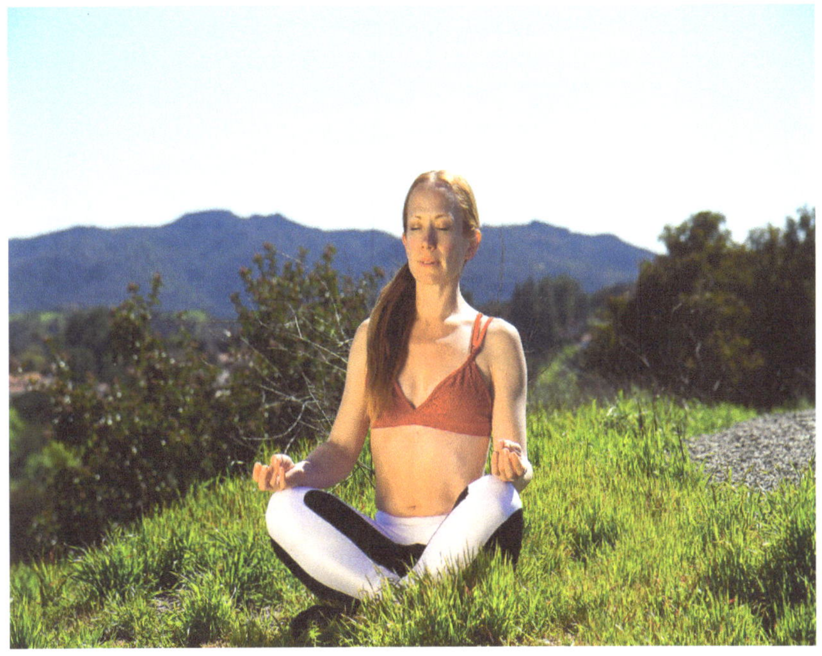

It's March now and about that time when our New Year's resolution workout routines are falling by the wayside. How many of you out there start the new year off with a workout routine or challenge? It could be yoga, training sessions, classes, you name it and then a week, a month, or 2 months in you fall off the wagon? HARD. It is important to think of your workout routine as part of your LIFE ROUTINE. That way, it's not just a quick fix, it's WHAT YOU DO. The best way to begin is to start with a baby step. We're all about, "I want it all now," and we throw ourselves into way too much too soon, with expectations that are too high to maintain and then we fall, HARD. What's the first baby step to this process, you may be wondering? SET YOUR MORNING WAKE UP CLOCK JUST 15 MINUTES EARLIER. I know, I know. The LAST thing you may want to do is get up a whole 15 extra minutes earlier, BUT if you do, you will be that much closer to feeling in tune with your body which means feeling not just good, but WONDERFUL in your body. Then you can and will WANT to progress into longer and more powerful routines that are REALISTIC AND ATTAINABLE over the LONG TERM of your life. So allow the FIRST THING YOU DO in your day to MOTIVATE AND INSPIRE YOU... it will be easier to maintain if you do it FIRST THING IN THE MORNING...here we go!

First: Bed spinal curl:
Roll out of that bed of yours and turn and face your whole body
towards it and reach out in front of you with your arms fully extended,
palms flat

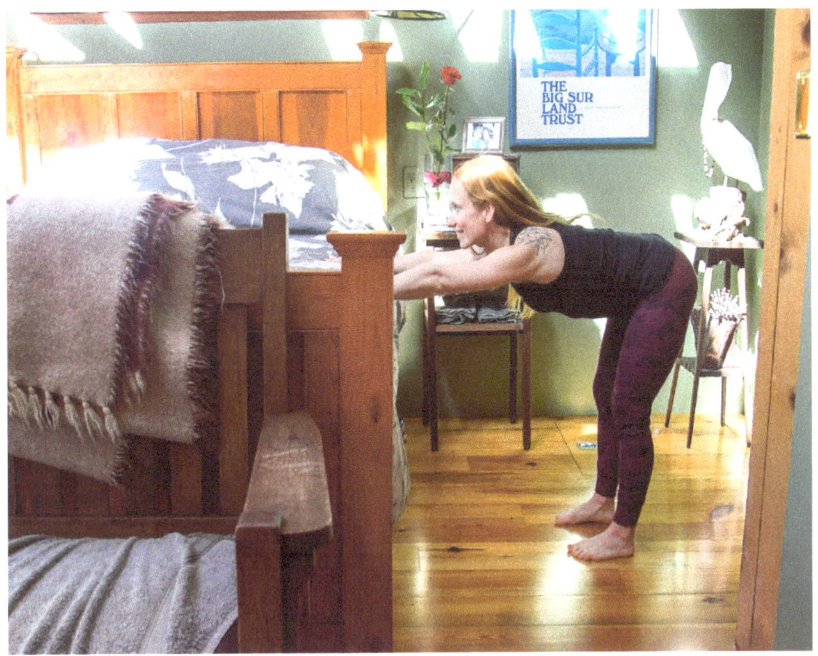

on the bed. Walk your feet back so that you toes are facing your bed
at a hip's distance and bend your knees a little since YOU JUST GOT
UP. BE GENTLE. Head relaxed, look at the floor and curl your spine,
like a cat might do.

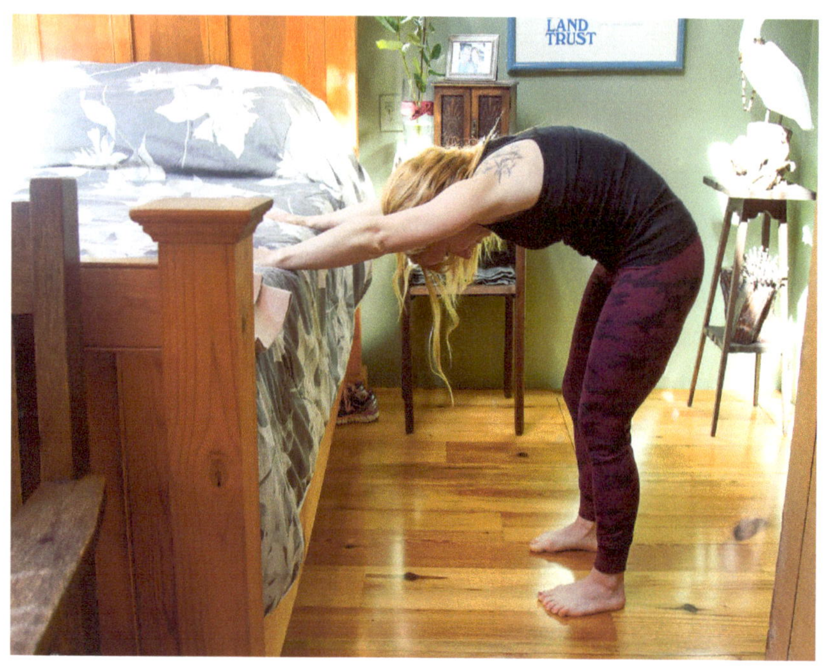

Then gently arch your back and look forward over your bed…this is cow pose. Inhale in the cow, exhale in the cat and start to become aware of your breath. Try a 5 count inhale through the nose and as you exhale for 5 counts through the mouth, engage your abdominal wall and your core with your deflation of your diaphragm. You are curling and extending your spine. AWESOME for your body! Try this about 6 times.

Second: Plank and pushups:
Draw your hands to the edge of the mattress now and make a plank position, rising up onto your toes and dropping your tailbone in line with your head so that you are flat as a board.

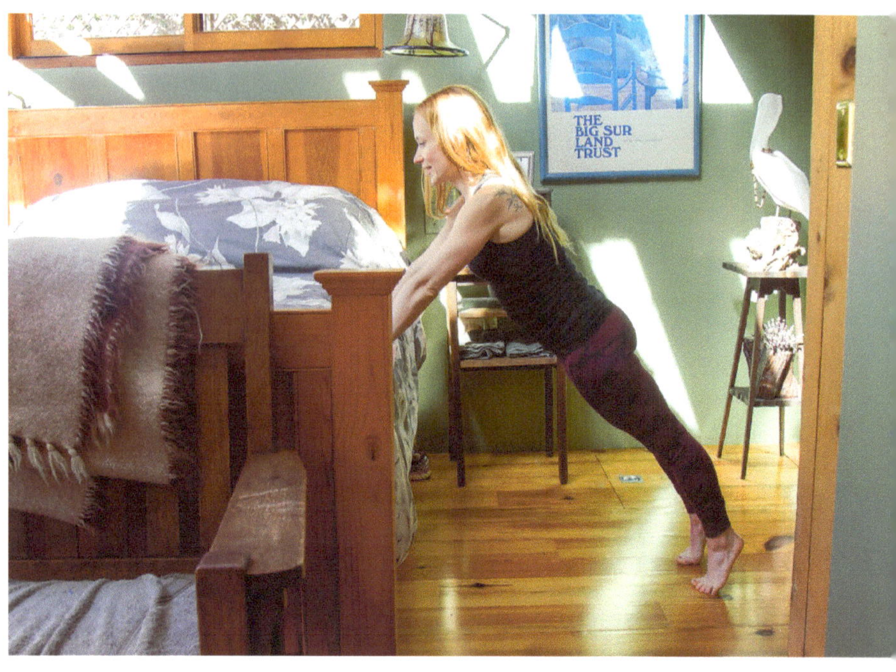

HOLD THE PLANK. As you breathe, now make your breath a little quicker. Breathe in and out in 2 count intervals and still activate that core! As you exhale, draw your belly button into your spine without changing your hip levels.

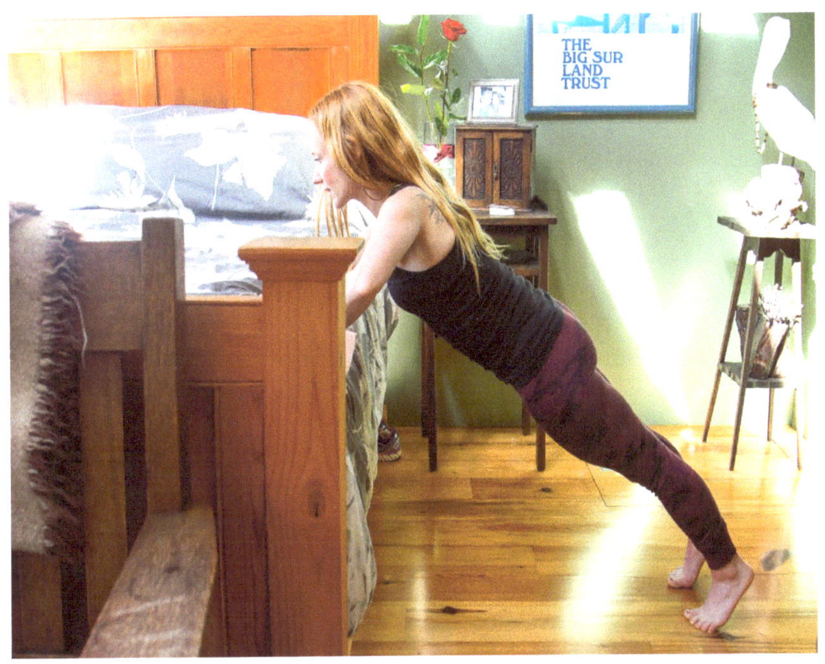

Now after about 4 breath cycles, do 10 push ups. Just take this shape and bend your elbows a bit and exhale as you push your body up. This is so good for our triceps, ladies! Oh, and your chests, men!

Third: Toothbrushing squats:
Now as you are brushing your teeth, stand with your feet facing
forward at a hip distance and squat, just like you are sitting in a
chair...

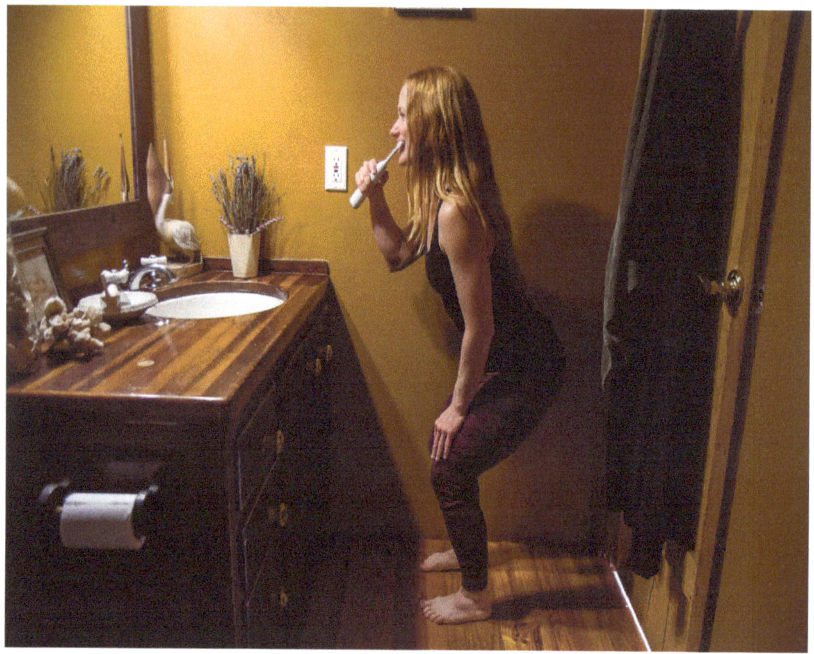

you want to stick your hips out, like you're going butt first into that
chair and hold it there for a breath. As you exhale, press down
through your feet and feel your gluteus maximus (largest butt
muscles) engage, all the while lengthening your spine.

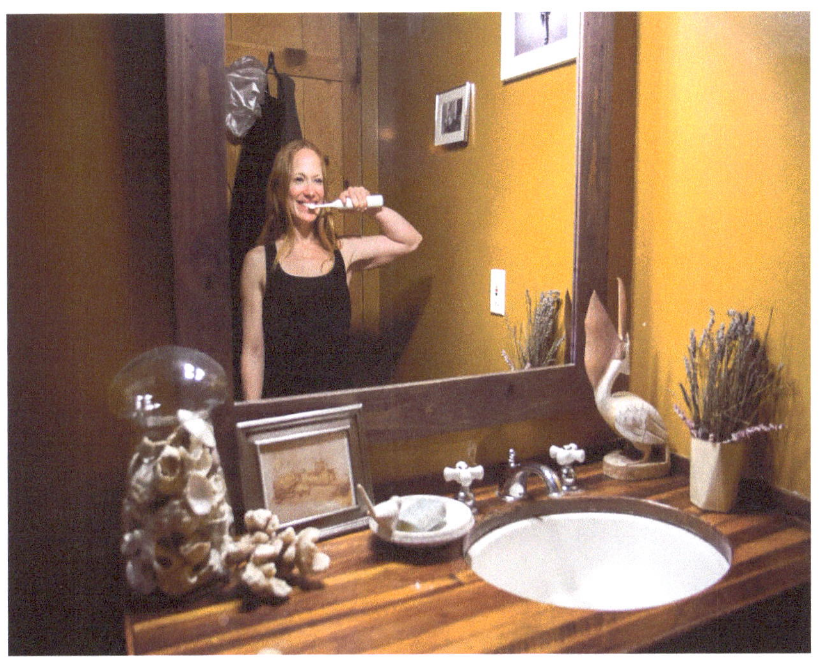

Do this while brushing about 8-10 reps….this will also improve your dental hygiene! **Interval addition if you're ready:** Try adding a jump in the air, but only if you're ready. This will give you an added high intensity interval, but make sure you land in that squat!

Fourth: Making coffee lunge/lift/balance:
You're in the kitchen now and whatever you make, be it breakfast, coffee, or tea it's time for some balance and a little more leg shaping! I make coffee the old school way, in a French press so I do these in the kitchen! You are going to stand with your feet facing forward, at a hips distance (sound familiar)?

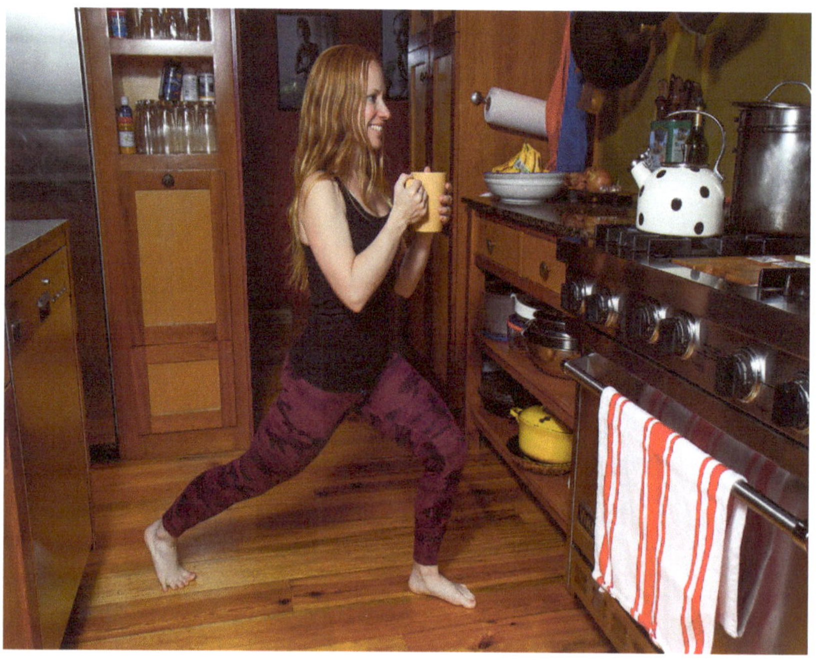

Take one leg back into a big lunge while staying on the ball of that foot and keep it parallel and then as you exhale think about engaging the supporting leg's glute muscles as well as your core and lift that lunged leg up in front of you, balancing on your supporting leg.

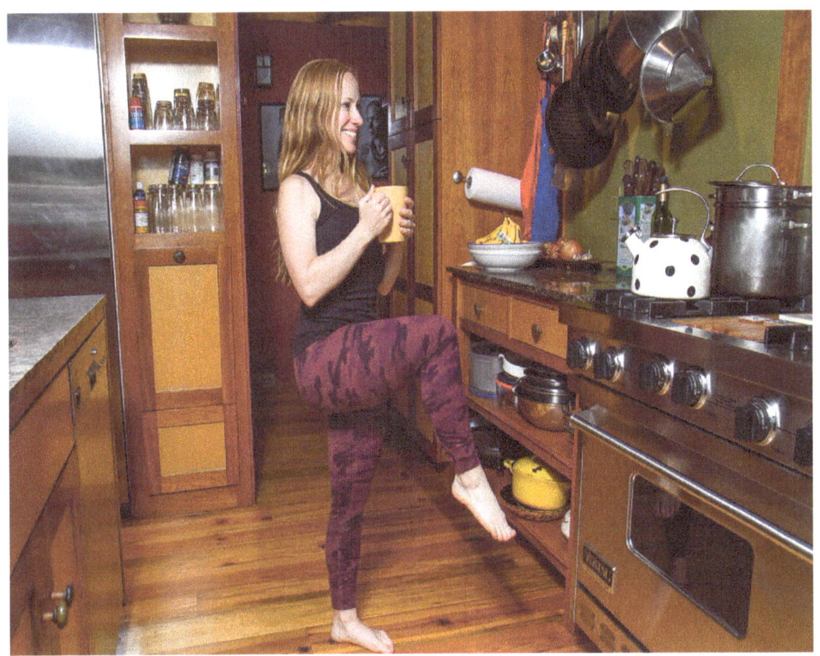

If you fall, who cares, you're doing it and that's what matters! You won't always fall. Do the same leg for 5 reps, then switch to the other leg. You'll probably notice one side is easier than the other, an added bonus to strengthening the symmetry of your body! However long it takes you to make your breakfast is the length of this exercise.
Interval addition if you're ready: After the lunge leg lift on one side, add a jump down to the floor,

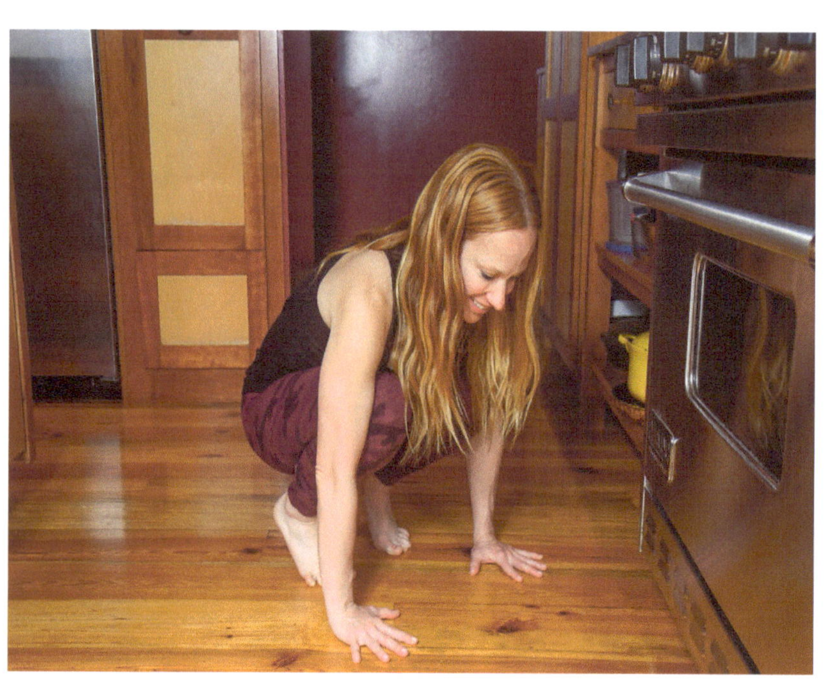

then a pop out into a plank,

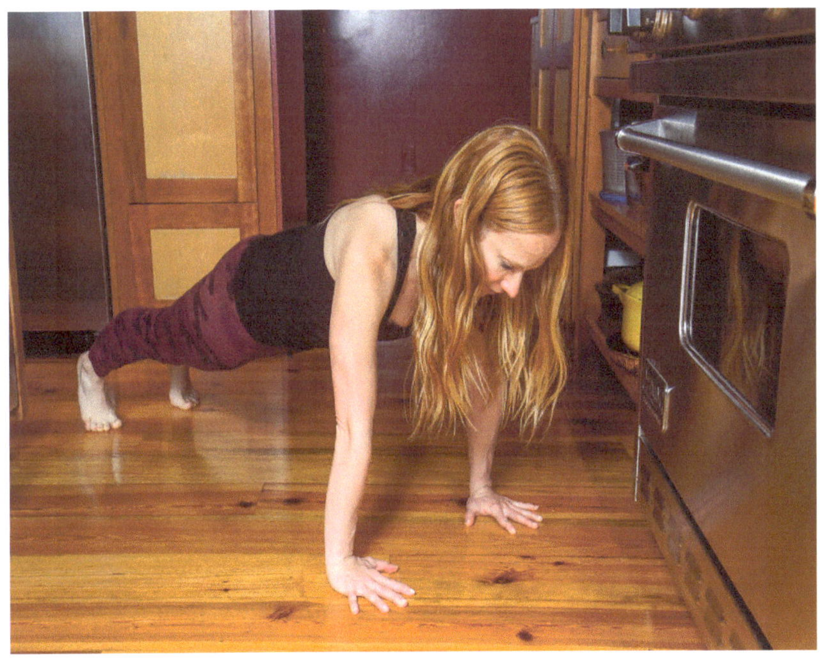

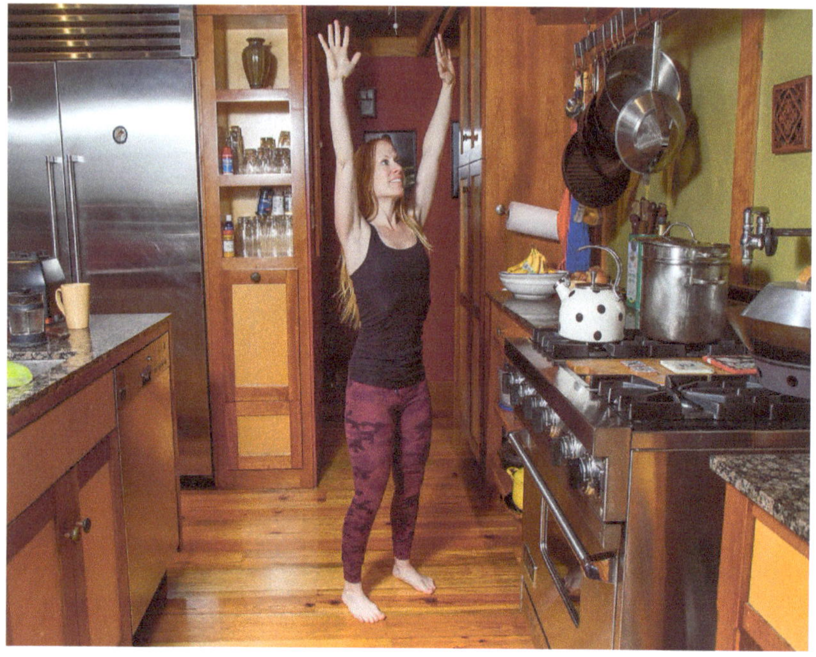

This is called a Burpee! Repeat on the other side, beginning with the lunge/lift/balance.

Fifth: After your shower tricep dip/figure 4 stretch combo:
As you're getting dressed lets get back to your arms. The side of the
bed or something lower works for this exercise. Place your hands
under your hips, fingers facing forward and walk your feet and body
out away from the bed or bench so that your arms are holding your
weight.

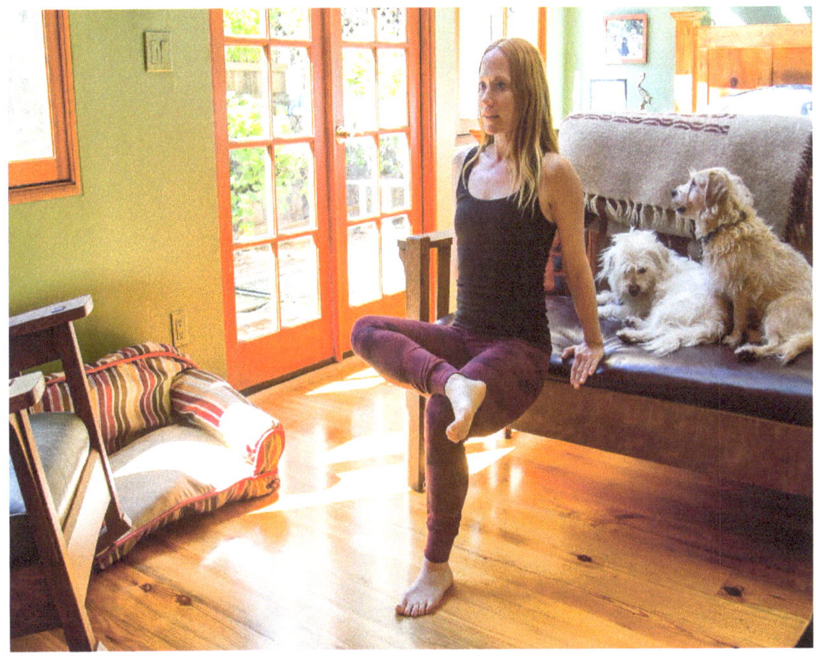

Bend your knees, lowering your pelvis and bend your arms, then
straighten for a tricep dip. Exhale as you push yourself back up to the
starting position, which will help you keep your core working to
support this exercise.

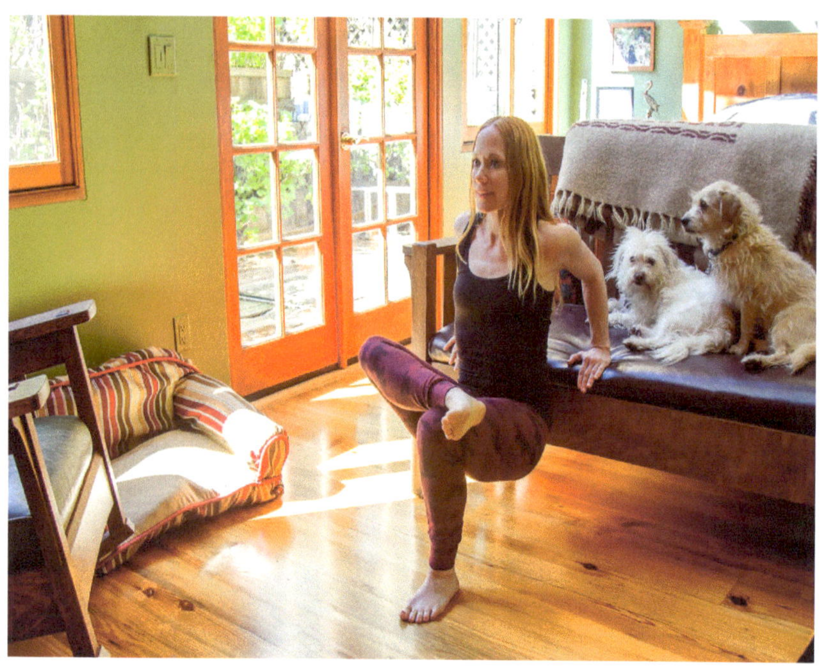

While you are dipping, do a FIGURE FOUR STRETCH. This is done by crossing an ankle over the other thigh, like a figure four. It feels great on the hips and is really good before you sit in that car for sometimes hours on end! It's also great to multi task your exercise. ☺ You will do about 10-15 dips, so try crossing right over left for 5-7 reps and then switch sides. **Interval addition if you're ready:** You will do 5-7 reps of this and THEN do 5-7 jumping jacks!

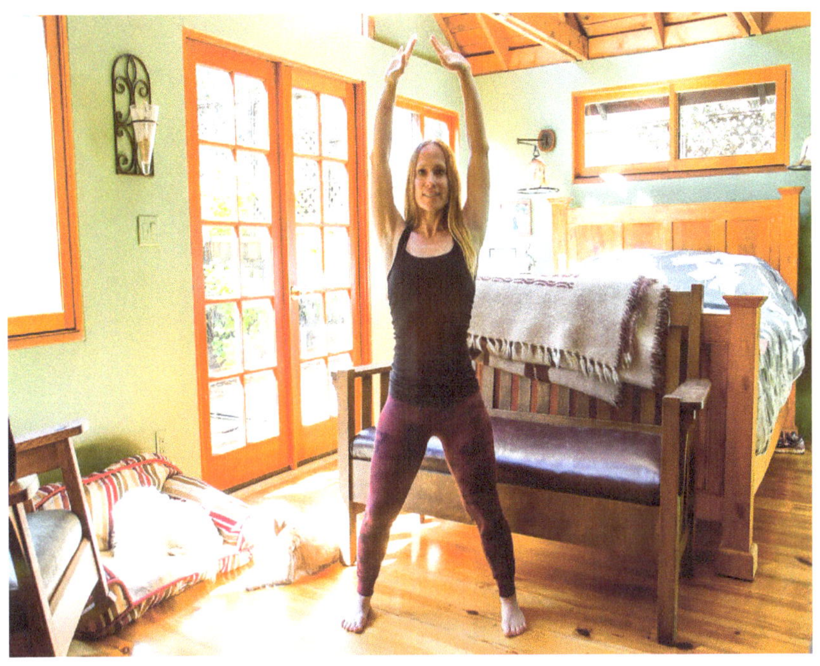

Repeat on the other side. You can do this whole series 3-4 times, depending on your speed. PS Your speed will improve with practice.

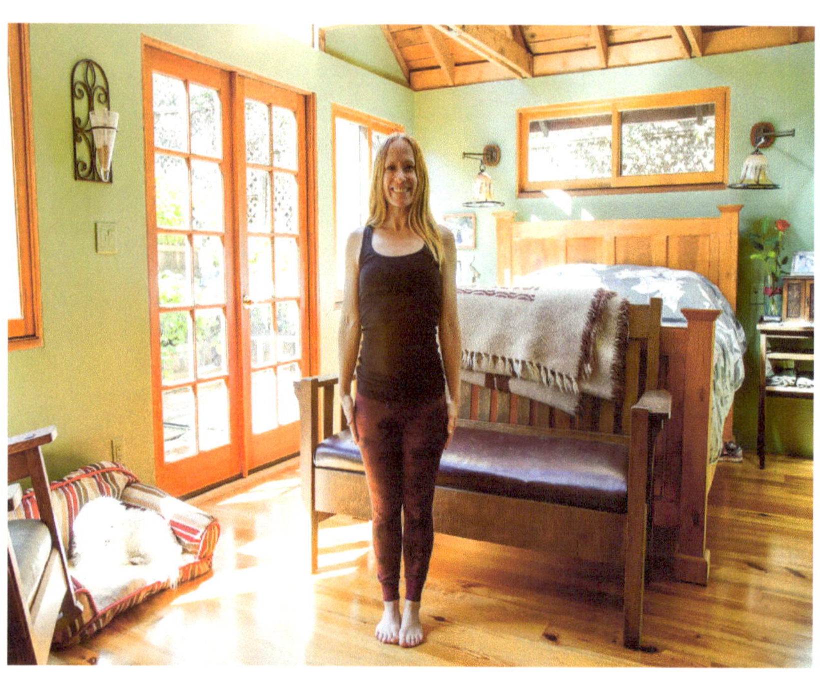

SIXTH: Nature breathing meditation
I know, you think I've already made you late and there's NO WAY this is only taking an extra 15 minutes, BUT I've timed it, so I know it can be done. You'd be surprised too at how much time you waste standing around! We've been doing MOST of these exercises while performing other daily routine activities, so just TRY IT! NOW, back to our sixth step. This can only take up 2 minutes of your time so feel free to set your timer on your phone and then DO NOT LOOK AT YOUR PHONE FOR THAT 2 MINUTES. Breathing, centering, and focusing your intentions for your day are of vital importance to creating success and fierceness in your being. I also believe that being in nature is really important. I know that some of us do not live in places that allow us to relax in nature, SO here's another way to achieve the same type of feeling… SIT NEXT TO YOUR PET.

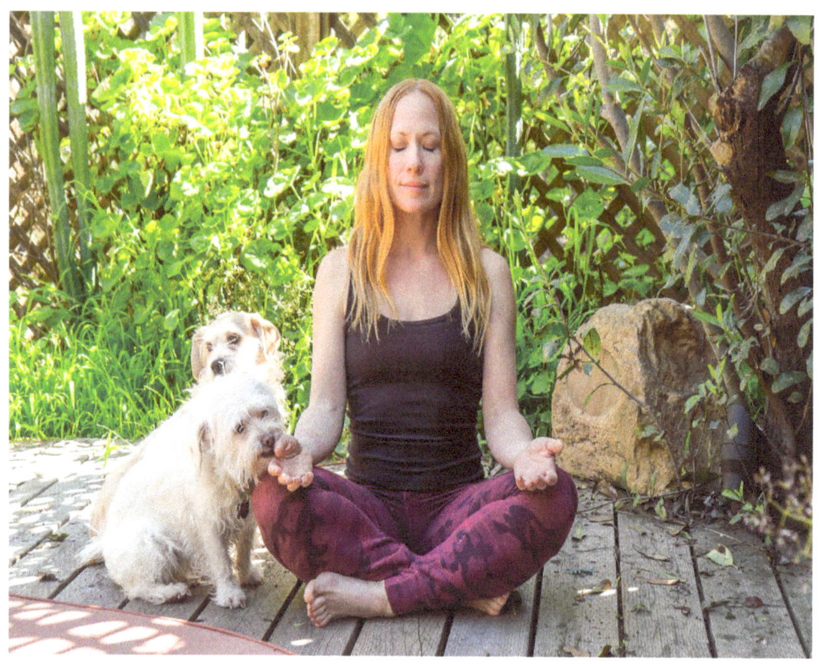

Your energy will calm them too eventually, so just take charge of your focused intentions. IF you do not have a pet or a great outdoor spot, find your most comfortable safe place in your house or apartment...maybe it is near a window and get as comfortable as you can on the ground, floor, or chair if you need and close your eyes. Allow your senses to explore what's happening around you and focus first on your breath. You don't need to breathe fast or slow, just allow your breath to become natural in your being. If you are feeling tension in any particular spot of your body, direct your energy to that spot and try to let it go. It may, it may not, but it's about the act of trying without forcing it. Try that inhale through the nose for a 5 count breath, and exhale through the mouth for a 5 count breath I asked you to do that at the beginning during our plank holds on the bed, remember? The counting will help slow your breath, create more lung-power and control, and help you focus your energy.

Now you're ready for your day. You have not exactly completed a crazy intense workout I know, BUT you have gotten your body to move. You completed the first baby step of getting up 15 minutes earlier in order to create body awareness, focus, and intention. Now you feel good in your body. If you find these few movement exercises to be easy to maintain after some time, THEN you are ready to take it the next level… and I've included some examples of adding high intensity interval moves above. Congratulations. You started somewhere that can only lead you ANYWHERE from here.

MOVE WELL, EAT WELL, BE WELL,
GINGER DANIELS Functional Fitness
Wellness Coach/Movement Specialist

Smoothie Recipes

-These recipes have ingredients with many incredible health properties! I have included a few examples of their benefits below so you know what and why you're putting them into your body…

Kale Power Morning Smoothie
-2-3 pieces of kale
-1 banana
-3 dates
-handful of beet greens
-1 scoop of brown rice protein powder-unflavored
-1 tsp turmeric
-1 tsp cinnamon
-1 tsp maca root powder, organic
-1/2 cup nonfat plain greek yogurt
-1 tbsp peanut butter
-1 cup unsweetened almond milk

Kale and beet greens are excellent sources of iron, especially good for those on a vegetarian diet. Banana has potassium, dates are a natural sugar for taste. Brown rice protein powder that is low in carbs, high in protein, and has low glecemic numbers is a great source of protein. Turmeric helps to act as an anti inflammatory, while cinnamon helps to balance your insulin levels. Maca helps to balance hormone levels, AND gives you a natural boost. Non fat plain greek yogurt is high in protein, low in fat, and has probiotics the body needs. Peanut butter is a great mood enhancer, and healthy fat. Almond milk has iron, vitamins, and minerals, and is great for those who are lactose intolerant.

Afternoon Re-energizer Smoothie
-1 small fuji apple
-1 avocado
-2 celery stalks
-1/4 cup chia seeds soaked in almond milk
-1/4 cup unsweetened cacao nibs
-1 tbsp almond butter
-1/2 pineapple
-1 cup coconut water
-1/2 tsp ginger root chopped

Apples have antioxidants and fiber, avocados have good healthy fat, celery is full of vitamin K, chia seeds have protein and omega 3 fatty acids, and having them in this form adds texture. Cacao nibs have mood stabilizers and flavonoids, almond butter has healthy fats and fiber, pineapple reduces swelling and has vitamin C, coconut water is full of potassium and electrolytes, and ginger has immunity boosting properties.

Evening Relaxing Smoothie
-1 cup unsweetened almond milk heated
-1/4 tsp nutmeg
-1 handful dried unsweetened cherries
-1 tsp raw honey
-1 tbsp pumpkin seeds
-1/2 cup blueberries

Almond Milk is an excellent source of calcium, nutmeg is for flavor and helps to relax you. Cherries also have relaxing properties. Honey is anti bacterial and anti fungal, pumpkin seeds have protein and tryptophan for sleep. Blueberries ward off heart disease and help brain function.